THE QUIET STORM

BY

Crystal Lynn

The Quiet Storm

THE QUIET STORM

BY

Crystal Lynn

Copyright © 2014 BY Crystal Lynn

Printed in the United States of America

The Quiet Storm

Acknowledgement

I want to thank my sisters and my mom for being there for me during this most challenging time in my life. Thank you Maria for always calling me at night just to ensure that I got home safely. I love you all.

The Quiet Storm

"From the brain and the brain only arise our pleasures, joys, laughter and jests, as well as our sorrows, pains, grief, and tears.... These things we suffer all come from the brain, when it is not healthy, but becomes abnormally hot, cold, moist or dry."

—**Hippocrates**

The Quiet Storm

The Quiet Storm

Table of Contents

The Quiet Storm

The Quiet Storm

It is unknown what causes certain diseases to occur, making your journey, when you have such a disease, an even more difficult one to travel. Uncharted waters, fear, anxiety, depression, and no one with whom you can compare the experience. Such rare conditions make situations even more challenging, to the point where you feel that you will be one of the unlucky ones, who, unfortunately, paves the way for other people.

"Every time he is going to be admitted, it hurts us so much; the pain gets worse with every admission." "The bright side is that he is getting closer to a full recovery – I hope."

Right before every admission, we were always very solemn and wanted to be by ourselves. If our grandson was visiting at the time, as soon as he would leave, Jose and I would immediately hold hands. It felt like what we thought was our pending doom. Words were not necessary.

The Quiet Storm

The Quiet Storm

Chapter One

Today I will visit mom to see how she is feeling. She is getting older, and slowly, her mental health is deteriorating, but not to the point that I can no longer hold a conversation with her. My mom is my best friend, and I confide all my deepest feelings to her. It's better to trust in her than in some of my so-called "friends."

I am in the living room with my mom, and we are chatting about everything that has been going on lately. I say to her that I have been feeling that Jose, my husband, is not going to live a long time. She asks me, "Why do you say that?" and I respond, "Something in my heart tells me that he is not going to live a long time." I don't know where this is coming from, but nevertheless I have a frightening feeling. As I tell her my fears, I hold

The Quiet Storm

back the tears. "It's just a feeling." I say to myself. "It's not happening."

I question myself because I have been known to have certain premonitions that have come true; it makes me skeptical, and I worry that my fears may become a reality. The latest thing that I dreamt about was having Clorox thrown at me from a window while I was standing at the bus stop. That was a weird dream I thought to myself.

Ironically the next day after having my dream, as I left my job at the end of my shift, I began to walk towards the bus stop. I noticed that there were some passersby looking upward because someone was throwing a liquid substance out the window. All of a sudden, a man yelled, "Someone is throwing Clorox." Wow! How can a dream be so precise regarding something so odd?

After leaving my mother's house, I do not

The Quiet Storm

continue to think about what I had told her earlier that day. I guess I am getting paranoid because we are getting older, and lately, we both have been feeling very sick.

The Quiet Storm

Chapter Two

It was October 10, 2013, when I was awakened by the sound of the phone – it was exactly 9:30 AM on a Thursday morning. I have developed quite a bad sleeping pattern after not working for six months due to my disability – going to sleep very late and waking up very late. Despite a long night of watching television, I sprang up from my sleep after hearing the phone ring.

The phone call was from the clinic where I was getting my physical therapy. The office was calling to let me know that my physical therapist would not be in for the day. Would I want another therapist? I had so many things to do that day that I opted to reschedule and catch up on my chores. I looked around and noticed that Jose was not home yet. It was customary for him to be home from work by 7:00 AM.

How odd that I had not heard anything from him by now, so I decided that I had to call him to find out exactly where he was. I called him on his cell phone, and he told me that he had passed out on the street and had been taken to the emergency room by ambulance. What caused this? Evidently, he would be in the emergency room for a number of hours. I asked Jose if he would be okay with me going to take care of my errands, and he responded yes.

Upon my arrival to the emergency room later that day, he seemed fine. He looked well, cranky as usual, and hungry because they had not fed him all day. It had now been about 10 hours since the ambulance had brought him into the emergency room, and still doctors had no explanation to offer.

He was very upset and wanted to leave. He said he was fine, and I believed him. Jose explained that he had gone into a supermarket in the morning to pick up some groceries and passed out right outside the supermarket. All this without warning, he said. How crazy… scary.

Apparently, a Good Samaritan helped him by calling an ambulance for him when he passed out. When he was picked up by an ambulance, he still had the groceries he had just purchased securely in his hands. Poor baby, tired and always thinking of his family. That is the kind of man he is – always putting others before himself.

We went home in a cab, and he rested for the rest of the evening; we always enjoyed being home with each other. That night, we left the emergency room on the premise that he would follow up with his primary doctor in three days, as he had a scheduled appointment already pending. He was feeling ok, and so I agreed.

The Quiet Storm

The doctor at the emergency room had made a point to emphasize the findings of this report, which made me curious why all the attention was being paid to this one area of the report. When I read the report, I noticed that it mentioned ischemic strokes. I gave Jose a copy of the CT scan report, and I attached a note like how a mother does with her child. I begged for the physician to please take his care seriously, as I could see his health was deteriorating.

In addition to passing out, Jose had lost about 20–30 lbs. in about two to three months' time without trying. His sleep deprivation was off the charts, and he had been looking very ill as well.

Monday rolled around, and as agreed, he went to the clinic to see his primary doctor. During the follow-up visit, Jose had showed his doctor the CT scan results from the day he passed out, as per the

The Quiet Storm

instructions of one of the treating physicians in the ER. Jose mentioned to the doctor about the ischemic stroke on the report, and she responded, "Where does it state that you had a stroke?" Jose replied, "Doctor, do you know how to read medical terminology?"

Despite sending a letter to his doctor regarding my concerns, Jose was never given the consultation to see a neurologist. In addition, the CT scan report stated to follow up with an MRI, and this was not addressed either. Apparently, she did not feel that this was not important enough either – she did refer him to see a cardiologist, though.

After returning home, Jose received a phone call from his primary doctor notifying him that his glucose level was extremely high – 600 mg/dl. High sugar levels could certainly put him in a coma. The doctor wanted him to come into the

The Quiet Storm

emergency room so he could be admitted due to the severity of his condition, so Jose agreed that he would go to the ER in the morning.

The Quiet Storm

October 13, 2013

To Whom It May Concern:

I am writing this letter because I am concerned about my husband, who presents to you today. He has been experiencing weight loss for the past couple of months without attempting to lose weight. In addition, he does not sleep well and has been looking and feeling weak the past couple of months.

I am also so puzzled that, in addition to him not feeling good, he is not getting the active care he urgently needs to find out what is the problem. Last time we left a message, it actually took one week before the doctor called us back – only because we called again.

This past Thursday, he blacked out after coming

The Quiet Storm

out of work. Not only was this scary, but what was even more frightening was the fact that it came without warning. After leaving work that day, he stopped by the supermarket, but the last thing he remembers is paying at the cashier. The rest is a blank spot until he regained consciousness.

Ever since Thursday, 10/10/13, he has been disoriented, hyperventilating, extremely emotional, and experiencing extreme tiredness. He has been resting and sleeping since coming home from the emergency room.

Doctor, I beg you to please evaluate him, as I have been watching him all these days and I am still very concerned regarding his health. In addition, he is thinking of going to work today for fear that he may lose his job. His health is of great concern to me, and I feel that he is not ready to return to work.

The Quiet Storm

I am attaching a copy of his release papers from the hospital where he was taken to when he passed out on 10/10/13.

If you have any questions, please do not hesitate to contact me immediately at xxx-xxx-xxxx.

The Quiet Storm

Chapter Three

Jose went to the hospital while I continued my last day of physical therapy, as my insurance was about to expire. Upon finishing my physical therapy that day, I quickly went to the area where he was being treated. When I got there, I saw him outside smoking a cigarette. Unbelievable that he was so sick, yet he would be outside smoking.

He was accompanied by a resident who was trying to convince him to go back inside the hospital. Infuriated at what I had just witnessed, I made him go back inside and lie down on the stretcher that he had been in since he'd arrived earlier that day. As soon as he took his place, the security officers approached us. Apparently the security staff was called in because he had gone outside the hospital premises. Jose was so upset by this, but we managed to speak to officials so they could back off. However, they did assign a nurse to watch over him.

He was admitted and released the next day. He would have to try to control his diabetes and diet so he could get his sugar level under control. I never thought that I had to intervene, so as usual, I tried not get involved; I did not think I had to.

Jose went to a couple of follow-up appointments after his initial visit with his primary doctor following the syncope episode. Finally, on one visit to the internal medicine department, his primary doctor was not there, and he was assigned to another physician, who finally gave him a referral to see a neurologist.

That day, I remember, he was at his doctor's visit when I called him on his cell phone to ensure that he had received a referral for a neurologist. As

The Quiet Storm

soon as he told me that the doctor had given him the referral, I called the neurology department to schedule an appointment for the neurologist; the next availability they had was for February 2014. I took this date in the meantime, but I had to work on getting something much sooner. This appointment was too far away for someone with such serious issues to have to wait for.

I asked the associate who answered the phone if there were any exceptions to getting an earlier appointment, and he responded yes, but that the patient had to have been to the emergency room recently due to passing out or stroke.

In the meantime, I tried to get in touch with the primary doctor by leaving several messages. I had to launch an official complaint with the patient services department against his doctor because we had not been able to communicate with her since

The Quiet Storm

leaving a message almost a month before. I filed another complaint. This time, I went on the Internet and filed a complaint with the Joint Commission, as I was so worried and desperate that I had to move heaven and earth.

Once I had filed an official complaint regarding the severity of needing to see a neurologist as soon as possible, we got a call with a date for early December 2013. Getting this earlier date was great, yet we still had not received a return call from his primary doctor. This neurology appointment was vital, as this doctor would be the one, according to the medical doctor, to give Jose the referral for the MRI that had been suggested as being necessary by the CT scan results. Time was crucial, and we had spent at least two months before seeing a neurologist.

The Quiet Storm

Chapter Four

Jose did not take much time to recuperate. In fact, an opening became available for a managerial position at the place where he was working. It had only been about a week and a half since he'd passed out in front of the supermarket after leaving work. However, Jose went back to work immediately because he felt that he needed to take care of his family. I was on disability, and he was trying to be a good provider.

He decided to go for this opportunity and began working the shift where a managerial position had become available. I was not sure if this was the right move, and I was not happy that he would take this role on. He looked so happy going to work every day, so I hoped that this would cheer him up. I had to ease up a little and let him be.

The Quiet Storm

One day while Jose was getting ready for his new job, I was observing him as he was standing in front of the mirror admiring himself. Right behind him was a figure of a young man who resembled our son. The strange thing about this was that our son was not home at the time. This figure was a little taller, his hair pushed back and two shades lighter. I said to myself, "This must be our son who we had lost two years before we had our only son." I watched him as he too was standing right behind Jose in front of the mirror. He then turned left and went right into my son's room. It was the second time I had ever seen him - the first being when he died as I held his little hand.

Day after day, he went to work and seemed to have an influx of emotions, both happiness and confusion. He was embarrassed because the job required him to count large amounts of money,

The Quiet Storm

which somehow had become a significant challenge.

Jose had always counted large amounts of cash, as he has always worked in retail and was used to such tasks. We had even owned a gift shop a couple of years before, so this should have been a piece of cake. However, it now seemed that this was a problem; and it was a big problem because this was vital to the job duties of the managerial position.

He trained for two weeks and began to feel he could not do this job. One of the managers even offered to come in on the weekend just so he could have one-on-one time with him to go over everything the job required. The senior manager was practically on the verge of tears seeing Jose's inability to train adequately due to the confusion. Jose was feeling embarrassed, and I reassured him

The Quiet Storm

that he had not taken enough time to recuperate after everything he had experienced. I felt he did not take enough time for his health issues, and most importantly, he had not seen the neurologist.

Despite the inability to continue in the administrative role, he continued to work and went back to his former shift to resume his position. Wishing he could go somewhere else, he stayed and became furious and resentful of his co-workers. This was not necessarily unjustified; he just wanted everyone to do what they were being paid for. He was always on time, and punctuality was a problem amongst his co-workers.

I suspected that there was something wrong with Jose. He was never much of a people person, but Jose was becoming increasingly angry and bitter. At times, he was just so angry that I thought his head was going to explode.

The Quiet Storm

The holidays are here, and as always, I began the routine I have every holiday: putting up the Christmas lights and decorations; creating a fireplace background for my tree to stand in front of; carefully picking decorations that go under the tree, such as glittery bags, bows that light up, etc.; going out on snowy or stormy days just to pick up the right kind of garland because I was so engulfed in the holiday spirit; and enjoying traditional foods such as pasteles, ham, turkey, roast pork etc. Oh, the joy of Christmas!

I wrote a Christmas poem, as I love all of the holidays beginning with Halloween and going right up until Easter, including birthdays and all occasions where I can decorate. The colors and warmth that these days bring out in people is priceless!!

The Quiet Storm

BELIEVE

To believe is to look to things we cannot see – we
call it faith.
Faith is believing that one day we will get what
God has planned for us.
Our world is filled with the belief that if we have
faith, we can achieve all that is wonderful and pure.
The happiness that the holidays bring,
when perfect strangers greet each other just because
it's no wonder they call it "the season of giving."
Our reflections of what should be
inspires us to give to those less fortunate.
The smile Christmas lights can bring, not only light
up the bulbs, but our faces as well.
For a moment, it's as if mankind is in a snow globe
all its own, forgetting all its sorrows – frozen in
time.
You have to believe in the spirit of Christmas.

The Quiet Storm

Jose had been going to the hospital quite a bit since he'd passed out in front of the supermarket during that cold October 2013 morning. However, he finally got to see a neurologist and was given a referral for an EEG and an MRI of the brain, which was scheduled the day after his upcoming family reunion.

Shortly before Christmas, Jose fell down once more when he got out of work, just as he was exiting the grocery store. He was in so much pain but did not go to the emergency room immediately; he ended up going a couple of days later due to the severity of the pain. The X-ray showed that he had fractured his ribs, and this pain was going to last a few weeks. It seemed like nothing was going good for him lately.

Sadly, we would not be playing the "That's My Grandfather" game any time soon. This is where I grab Jose and hug him so tightly, making it

The Quiet Storm

impossible for my grandson Dylan to get in between us, which drives him crazy. It brings the three of us so much happiness to play this game. It's the simple things.

Chapter Five

Jose comes from a large family. There is a total of ten siblings: six sisters and three brothers. The past couple of years, they had been getting together for certain holidays – July 4th seems to be a big one. Their reunions were usually about six hours away which made it difficult for us to attend.

However, this year the family gathering would be closer to us, and Jose's sister and brother-in-law picked him up early in the morning. Before they headed to the reunion, they stopped by one of the bakeries used quite often by my sister to pick up some desserts. The bakery was so popular that it was only 6:30 AM and they were almost out of pastries. I was happy that he went to spend time with his family. Many times when he was invited, he said he would go and never followed through,

The Quiet Storm

but this time he did. He called me quite frequently that day.

I think he was not very comfortable there, as he rarely spent much time with them. Nonetheless, I am glad he made an effort to attend.

The next day, Jose went to have the MRI that we had been waiting for since he'd passed out back in October 2013. Unfortunately, when he got to the hospital and was registered, the hospital staff deemed it unsafe to do an MRI and did an X-ray as an alternative. This was due to an incident that Jose had been involved in many years before when he was very young – he had been shot in the head and removed the bullet himself.

After Jose came home from the hospital, I noticed that he was very irritable, although he claimed he was happy. He was upset at me for some reason. He was mad that I had made him

The Quiet Storm

attend the family reunion. He went through different motions, as if this gathering had put him in some sort of tailspin. He seemed more than upset, yelling like a madman.

Lately, he had been so aggressive and hated everyone. He was never much of a people person, but he was always honest with his feelings, something that most people did not appreciate.

Despite having a rocky start at adolescence , that way never stuck with him. It was almost as if that life had never existed. Jose was an entirely different man; the only things that remained were the memories of the poor choices he'd made during that time. I guess this could be attributed to his upbringing in the church. He had been raised attending church on a regular basis with his mother and siblings, even becoming the president of the juvenile association at the Calvary Christian Church in New York City.

The Quiet Storm

That day, he just was so mixed in emotion. As I am thinking about it now, he has seen so much violence growing up. The people who he has encountered, the stories, are just endless – even after thirty years, he still surprises me with far-out stories.

I remember when he told me about the story of the Jamaican woman who had been scorned by someone whom she was dating. Jose was about nine years old at the time, when a crazed woman passed by him carrying a scalding bowl of oatmeal with a little something special inside. She tapped Jose on the shoulder and told him, "Look at this, man, watch what is going to happen." The woman then threw the hot bowl of oatmeal at the face of the man who had scorned her, and the man began to howl in pain as he tried to get the oatmeal off his face. He raised his hands to his face, as he began to bleed. The woman had thrown crushed glass in the

The Quiet Storm

mix of scalding oatmeal.

This is a memory that should not be in anyone's brain – no matter the age!

I believe the night with the family did something to the depths of his brain's subconscious. For the life of me, I did not understand why he was upset. He continued to carry on about how I'd made him go to the family reunion, and he did not want to go to his family reunions anymore. I was so baffled; I had no clue what went wrong. Even while I was filing some of my papers away, he slapped my portable filing system closed. He seemed belligerent. Since he continued to argue and came close to me in a menacing way, I grabbed his hand and put my nails to his throat. This was not the way we were used to being with each other.

This was so out of character of him. He loved and respected his brothers and sisters so much.

The Quiet Storm

Chapter Six

It has been three months since Jose passed out in the street after coming out of work and going to the supermarket. Lately, he has been feeling very sick; I have told him that it is time he stopped working. He is so proud, and he feels that he cannot quit his job while I am in need of his support the most. I feel so sorry for him, as he goes to work every day so sick. He is so sleep deprived – usually, he might not even get three hours of rest after a long day at work.

Jose has been forgetting so many details this past couple of weeks. For example, he does not remember what he is supposed to be doing each day, whether he is supposed to be working, what time it is, etc. It seems like he's been struggling every day. I never thought that this struggle was

The Quiet Storm

anything more than usual malaise. I think he needs a vacation. I tell him, "Don't forget when you get to your job, let your boss know that you need some time off – at least two weeks of vacation." Day after day, he goes to work and does not let the bosses know that he wants some time off.

I worry when he goes off to work; he has been so unhappy lately. He has been telling me that working is becoming a struggle because he forgets things at his job. This forgetfulness is cause for alarm – I have no idea what is going on. There seems to be something awfully wrong with Jose. Passing out, feeling sick, lack of sleep, extreme chills, not feeling better even after sleeping for hours, the headaches, the anger, depression, anxiety, panic attacks, nodding out, etc.

I feel like I have to get more involved with his medical care. I notice that he is struggling with his sugar levels. The sugar levels continue to be out of control and his behavior lately is cause for alarm. I am getting apprehensive and have reason to believe he is not taking his medication as prescribed. I look into his pill dispenser and see that his pills are not set up correctly. In addition, he takes insulin for diabetes, which I am sure he is not doing as he should be either.

In the middle of all this confusion, I assign myself caregiver and begin to ensure he is taking his medication properly, as he seems very sickly and cannot continue to deteriorate. I start getting up early in the morning to make sure he does everything as he should. I make him breakfast and send him off to bed, as he is very sleep deprived. I have even prohibited Jose from picking up our grandson Dylan, who we pick up every weekend. I am afraid that Jose will pass out and tumble onto the subway tracks. He has been so tired lately, and

The Quiet Storm

resting does not seem to be working for him.

33

The Quiet Storm

One weekend after Dylan had gone home, Jose began to develop extreme chills and to shake uncontrollably. I offered to take him to the hospital; instead, he opted to go into the shower. I brought along my iPod to document what was going on. I typically do not take any recording devices to the bathroom, but as Jose began to shiver, his body began turning purple all over. I thought this could be useful when he went to the doctor.

This was such a concern because of the dark shade of purple he was turning, but he explained that this had happened to him before. I had been around him for thirty years – I had never witnessed this, ever!

After his bath, we settled in the sofa. He had

been having bad headaches lately, so I began to massage his neck and his temples to see if I could make him feel better. He was so upset at the way he had been feeling lately. He began to let me know of his wishes in the event of his death. We talked about him wanting me to find a new love interest. He expressed that he thought it was unfair that I would stay by myself at such a young age. Lying down opposite to him, all I did was cry silently as he spoke. Little did I know that it would be the beginning of many tears to come.

Monday, January 27, 2014, Jose seemed ok until I noticed that he was testing his blood sugar level and that it was excessive – 479 mg/dL to be exact. I had been noticing that this was an issue lasting longer than it should be, and so I decided that I should intervene in order to help him out. So I began to go through his pill dispenser and syringes, gathering them up. I would ensure that things were

The Quiet Storm

done properly, and then I would turn everything over back to him once I felt it was safe to do so.

The problem with the high sugar level had been going on for months, since October 2013, when he'd passed out in the street early in the morning exiting the supermarket. This was alarming because high sugar levels over long periods of time can be extremely dangerous.

I also noticed he had been getting to work late without notifying his job of his tardiness. He was disillusioned with his job, hated his co-workers, and was so angry about everything. This behavior seemed a little off to me. I would say to myself, "His brain is going to explode one day." Everything about Jose was making me nervous.

What was even more bizarre was that Jose seemed to be having very serious panic attacks lately; this started about early December 2013. He had even gone to the psychiatrist to get a prescription for anxiety and panic attacks, yet he continued to experience high anxiety. So, in addition to the prescription for anxiety he'd received at the clinic, I also got him a natural remedy for anxiety, hoping that this would help him. As I look back now, there was an occasion before December 2013 when he had a panic attack on the bus and had to get off because he was feeling extreme anxiety.

Watching him go to work was heart breaking, especially with everything he had been going through, mainly because he had such severe sleep deprivation (something he'd always had but gotten much worse). This seemed like a lethal combination. All this odd behavior mixed with intense anxiety, mixed emotions, illness, and confusion.

The Quiet Storm

How would this all end?

The Quiet Storm

Chapter 7

January 30, 2014, Jose came home from work unusually late. As soon as I heard him come in, I opened my eyes. He seemed as if he was not feeling well. I also noticed that he had gotten home about two hours late; he was usually home by 7:00 AM. I asked him why did he get home so late, and he said he'd gotten confused and ended up at the apartment where he had lived in with his mother and siblings. He'd then realized that he should not be there and heard the voice of his mother, who had died thirteen years ago, telling him to go home.

I was so concerned over this odd behavior. What possessed him to go to the old neighborhood? Why was he communicating with his dead mother?

I got up early in the morning to ensure that he took his medications, ate breakfast and went to sleep at a reasonable time. After breakfast was served, he settled into the bedroom to finish eating while I sat in the living room. I had been on disability for months, so I had nowhere to go during the day. I heard him snoring, and it made me happy — it was like music to me ears. It was a little after 10:00 AM when he had fallen asleep. I tried to keep the house quiet so he could sleep peacefully.

All of a sudden, I heard sounds from the bedroom: odd noises, like the sound of aah, aah. The sounds seemed unfamiliar to me. I ran into the room, and I saw Jose face down in the bed with his breakfast alongside him. He sprang up from the bed, sat up, and began to clap like when a baby sees its mother. I asked him, "Are you ok?" He smiled and looked as if he were deranged. He stood up, took my hand, and began to kiss it as he tried to go out the bedroom door. I cupped his face in my

40

The Quiet Storm

hands and asked him, "What's wrong?" His speech was incomprehensible, aah, aah, aah. "Jose," I asked him again, "What's wrong?" I saw his right arm go limp and then the rest of his body started to go down as well. I gently lay him on the floor and began to search for the cordless phone I had put away earlier that morning so he it would not disturb him.

I found the phone and got back to Jose, who was lying on the floor. He began to convulse while I called 911. His body was shaking back and forth, and he began to snore very loudly as I was speaking to the 911 operator. The 911 operator was so astonished by the fact that he was seizing and snoring. I had never seen anyone that I cared for, or anybody else, have a seizure. I told the operator that he might be having a stroke, given the fact that back in October, the CT scan showed he'd had ischemic strokes.

The Quiet Storm

I remained calm while I waited for the ambulance to arrive — it arrived pretty quickly. As a matter of fact, there were two ambulances that were dispatched to my address. This was probably due to the fact that I stated there was a possibility of him having a stroke. One ambulance had a medical doctor; however, she had nothing to do with him. It seemed almost as if she was upset because he was not having a stroke. She stood by the doorway while the technicians did all the work. The first technician recognized him right away. He said, "This is my patient. I remember being flagged down by a group of people while I was on my way to another call. I remember him because he was holding two bags in his hands."

Jose had never known what had happened to him when he had left the supermarket that day. He never saw it coming.

The Quiet Storm

Jose was taken to the emergency room after being stabilized. I expressed that I wanted him to be taken to the hospital where he was getting treated, but the emergency medical technician did not feel he was stable enough to go the extra mile. Upon arrival at the hospital, they performed different tests on him. After about an hour, the results became available, and the doctor recommended that Jose be admitted to determine what caused the seizure. Jose was stubborn and did not want to be admitted into the hospital. The resident pulled me to the side and urged me to try to convince him to stay. She was concerned about the results of the CT scan of his brain. She asked him what year was it, and he responded, "2006." WOW! THIS WAS SO ALARMING.

Regrettably, Jose signed himself out against doctor's orders and my wishes. The doctor gave him a prescription for Dilantin and once again, we

The Quiet Storm

left on the premise that he would follow up with the neurologist next week. His treating hospital had already done an EEG on him in the neurology department where we had fought so hard to get an appointment at, and the results would be available by then. His medical history was in one area, and he preferred to wait to go to the hospital where he was being treated.

It had been a frigid and snowy season so far; the snowfall totals for that winter had made new records. We stepped outside, and I was nervous due to Jose discharging himself against hospital advice and still feeling ill. I held him tightly and bought us some deli sandwiches, as we began our way home. When we got home, he was so out of it, he just wanted to lie down. I asked him, "Are you ok?" and he responded, yes. He went into the shower and stood in there for quite some time. When he finished, he went right into the bed.

The Quiet Storm

After a few minutes, he got up and started to babble the way he had done earlier that morning right before he got his seizure. I said to Jose, "We have to go back to the emergency room because you are still not feeling well." I called my son to tell him that I had to take Jose back to the emergency room because it seemed as if he were going to have another seizure. I started to dress Jose and sat him down on the ottoman that is in front our bed. I placed pillows right in front of him just in case he fell forward – he was not saying much at all. He quickly jumped in the bed and covered himself. I asked him, "Jose, do you know who I am?" He smiled and went to sleep. What did this mean?

He fell asleep about 9:45 PM. I was so scared over the crazy day I had experienced that I just fell back on my sofa and cried. I thought to myself, I should contact his family... I called his brother

45

The Quiet Storm

Felipe, who is a doctor, and went over everything with him. I discussed everything from the moment he'd gotten home that morning and had the seizure, to the ER visit, the test results, right down to the point when I'd asked him if he knew who I was. We spoke for about two hours. He immediately said to me, "Carol, this is not good. This is a deadly disease." He repeated this to me several times. This phrase resonated in my brain over and over again. Felipe said he would call me in the morning to check on Jose.

As I sat down to think about what had happened to Jose that day, I was happy that the emergency medical technician who had taken care of Jose once before was able to tell me a little about what had happened on the October 2013 morning when Jose had collapsed in front of the supermarket. I could share the story with Jose when he got a little better. Small world.

The Quiet Storm

I stood in the living room all night long. I got down on my knees, and I prayed to God to help Jose. All I did was cry all night long, constantly opening the door to peek in on Jose, desperate to see how he would wake up. Was his memory gone?

Why didn't he just tell me who I was? Oh my God, the pain. I could relate to the expression, "heavy heart." My heart felt like it weighed about fifty pounds from all the pain I was going through.

I finally fell asleep about the time that Felipe said he would call to check on Jose. So before the phone would ring, I texted him to let him know that Jose was still sleeping and had not woken up all night. I would contact him later on during the day.

When Jose got up in the morning, I had never been so happy to see his big eyes open and look up at me. I asked him if he was okay, and he

The Quiet Storm

responded yes. I asked him, "Do you remember who I am?" and he said, "How am I not going to know who you are?" I asked him if I could hug him, and I wrapped my arms around him and began to cry uncontrollably. He said, "Oh my God, it must be bad."

It was Friday, and we stepped out to take care of a couple of chores that we needed to do. It was cold, and Jose was on super cranky. We got in a cab, and when he asked the cab driver the cost of the cab ride, he got irate. When we were coming back home after taking care of our errands, I saw the bus that passes by our house and we decided to get on. I went straight to the back of the bus and took a seat when I noticed that Jose had exchanged words with the bus driver.

They continued again just as we were exiting the bus, and I noticed that the bus driver was giving

The Quiet Storm

him the finger as we were walking away from the bus. When I saw what the bus driver was doing, I took a picture of the driver and the bus. The bus driver noticed what I had done and caught up with us, trying to offer an explanation regarding his actions. He explained that he was baffled that Jose was acting this way because they had always spoken to each other whenever Jose traveled on his bus route. My response was, "And you are no better." I did not report the driver.

When we got home, Jose was so exhausted and went straight to bed. It was only Friday, and his appointment was on Tuesday – it seemed like forever. He did not get up at all. I would have to get him up so he could eat. Every time he got up at night, I would rush to hug him, and of course, I would also start crying.

I noticed that, in addition to him feeling

The Quiet Storm

fatigued, sleepy, and unable to do anything for himself; he was also having problems remembering important things. For example, he did not remember that he'd had a seizure, and he couldn't recall the date, the time, the year, or where our grandson was. I did research on the Internet to see what goes on after a person has a seizure, but these symptoms should not still be going on. He should have moved past feeling this way. I read that some people even experience anterograde amnesia.

Since he was having problems with his memory and driving me crazy asking the date, I thought I would get an advantage over the situation. I wrote down the day of the week, the date, and the year on a piece of paper and posted it so that, when he asked me again, I could just direct him to where he should look. So when he asked me again, I said, "Look on the wall," and he responded, "Very funny."

The Quiet Storm

Finally, Tuesday arrived, and we went to his neurology appointment together. I explained to the doctor everything that Jose had been experiencing, and the doctor's recommendation was for him to be admitted into the hospital, but once again, he did not want to stay.

We went home, but he continued to feel terrible. He was still lethargic and unable to do anything for himself. By the next day, I put my foot down and said, "We are going to the hospital – this is not up for debate." While on my way to the hospital, I called and left a message for the neurologist to inform her that we were on our way to the emergency room due to Jose not improving at all. Whatever this was, it was not going away anytime soon.

He was admitted, and we hoped he could get the help he so desperately needed. He needed to be in

The Quiet Storm

the hospital, and I needed to get some piece of mind knowing that he was getting the necessary care. I could only do so much for him. This was something that we couldn't shake off, wait out, or treat at home.

As soon as he was admitted, he went into the neurology ward. The brain monitor was placed on him immediately, and they began to screen his brain activity. When I went to visit him, I was taken back when I saw his head all

wrapped up. I had never seen anyone in this situation ever. In the 30 years that I had been around Jose, I had never known him to have a seizure. All this was new to me. This meant that we would definitely have to make some major changes in our lives. He was still having problems with his memory, but not to the point where he would forget the important people in his life.

The Quiet Storm

When I got up in the morning, I called his brother Felipe to give him an update on the latest developments. Jose had had about 15 seizures during the night. Wow! This was worse than I could have imagined. The ironic thing about the EEG monitoring done on him back in January 6, 2014, was that it had registered as normal.

Jose's brother, Felipe, wanted the treating physician's telephone number so he could speak to him/her to get a perspective from a doctor's point of view. After he had spoken with the treating physician, we spoke for a couple hours, going over Jose's issues and how he needed to make some lifestyle changes. Jose had always had a problem with his sleeping pattern. Changing this had to be at the top of the list. Secondly, was his eating pattern. He needed to control his intake of food so he could stabilize his sugar

The Quiet Storm

level. I would be on patrol from now on! I also spoke to the doctor in charge, and she said he was stable, but it would get worse before it got better. Strangely, those words seemed to comfort me.

Jose was discharged from the hospital one week later, right before Valentine's Day. I was so happy that he was being discharged and that there were going to be major lifestyle changes for him. Of course, the house was decorated for Valentine's Day and had been since before the day he'd gotten his first seizure back in January 30, 2014.

I went to the pharmacy and sent Jose home to settle in while I waited for his new medications. During the short time I was separated from him, Jose was enjoying some of the goodies that were at home. Like I said, "Some things were going to change." We settled in for the evening, and it seemed that Jose's appetite had come back, as he was overindulging in his favorite foods constantly.

The Quiet Storm

A couple of times when I got up in the middle of the night, I would catch Jose eating. I told him this was not good for his health and advised him that he needed to stop this immediately.

I began to incorporate healthier options to our shopping list, replacing the junk food for things such as fruits, vegetables, and nuts. I ensured that he went to bed early so he could get the rest that he so desperately needed. I was already feeling responsible for buying the Halloween candy back in October 2013 that had elevated his glucose to dangerous levels. I would have to be a hard ass and get on his case. I did not enjoy being a nag. I always hated people who nagged or yelled. In this relationship, I was the mellow one, and Jose was the one who was always nagging.

Jose was a smoker, and I was not going to allow him to smoke either. Although he'd been given patches by the doctor, I decided he was going to

The Quiet Storm

quit "cold turkey." He was so sick already, and I was not about to start using patches to wean him off. A couple of times, he became resentful and said that I would not be able to do such a thing if I smoked. I had to remind him that I, myself, had stopped "cold turkey" when I smoked because I had become so sick and felt as if I was going to die. It took months before my health began to stabilize and I could finally breathe a little better. The terror of that night, when I could barely breathe, had kept me from ever putting a cigarette in mouth ever again.

I took notes regarding what I noticed about Jose from day to day – it was not good. I would make sure to go with him to his appointments because I could not rely on his judgment for two reasons: 1. His memory was in poor shape 2. He did not want to be admitted again and probably would not be honest with me.

The Quiet Storm

Chapter 8

Finally, the day for his follow-up appointment had arrived and, of course, so did another winter storm! It was so snowy that morning, but this appointment could not be missed. We bundled up and headed off to the neurologist. I made sure Jose was prepared to be in a winter storm.

When we got into the neurologist's office, I did all the talking. I read from my notes regarding everything that Jose was experiencing. I told the doctor he was having a lot of difficulty with regards to his memory, appetite, energy, and experiencing severe confusion. He was unable to tell me the year, month, date or even the season. The doctor went to meet with her superior, and when they came back together, they recommended that Jose be admitted once again.

The attending said, "I am going to admit you, but you look so handsome that no one is going to believe that you are sick." The reaction on Jose's face was hurt and pain. He did not want to be in the hospital any more than I wanted him in there, but this was not up for debate. Of course, I reminded him of all that he was going through, and he eventually agreed to be hospitalized. I was not going to go home and have to come back tomorrow in this blizzard because he was still not well. We needed to get to the root of this problem. The doctor sent us to the emergency room, and once again, Jose was admitted. It was now March 5, 2014.

Given that this time he was being admitted with a different concern, I thought the doctors would approach his care differently. This time the doctor was concerned with the problems with his memory. After two days of being in the hospital, I got a call from the doctor who was now overseeing his case. Dr. Ji Yeoun Yoo was asking me all types of questions, e.g., if he had traveled anywhere, how long had he been feeling this way, etc. I described to her how he had experienced such severe leg cramps that you could see the muscles contracting. It had been so intense that I had used my iPod to capture him in excruciating pain just in case it was significant to his care.

She expressed that she would like to see the video when I came in to see him. She told me that she suspected Jose had what is known as "limbic encephalitis." She went over all the test that were going to be done on him, e.g., spinal tap, CT scan and bloodwork. She also mentioned that she wanted to do an MRI despite the controversy regarding possible bullet fragments in his brain.

Did I mention taking a trip to hell? This would

The Quiet Storm

have been a picnic compared to how I was feeling right now. I felt like I was in the abyss and was not going anywhere, any time soon. In addition to Jose going through all this, I was feeling so sick that day. I had a headache, an ear ache, a toothache, and an abscess in my mouth too. Boy, I had to take one thing at a time, or I was going to lose it.

First things first – I needed to get to the dentist right away. I had been calling different locations to see if there was a dentist willing to see me that day. Then I finally got a call back. I headed to the dentist's office first before I went to see Jose at the hospital. I called his nurse to let her know what was going on with me and went to take care of my dental issue.

Just as I had gotten to the hospital later on that day, they were just finishing up the spinal tap that needed to be done on him. He had been such trooper so far during this whole ordeal. He had either managed to remain calm or was just too sick to complain. I asked to have the doctor paged so that I could show her the video. When she came into Jose's hospital room, I showed her the video, and once again, she went over everything that they would be doing for Jose's treatment plan.

While the transporter took Jose to have his X-rays and CT scan done, I began to eat a hot dog that I'd brought with me. When Jose was brought back up to the floor, he was taken to the other side of the hallway while I just sat there in his room waiting for him to return. The transporter entered the room and began to remove everything that belonged to Jose. It was almost as if I was invisible. Infuriated by this action, I asked to speak to the administrator on duty. This was outrageous!

The Quiet Storm

They were placing him in a semi-private room due to a patient who had arrived who was actively having seizures and needed a private room. The hospital staff attributed this mistake to lack of communication and were very apologetic about the mix-up. I was not there to fight. I just wanted Jose to get better, but this upset me so much, as we were already going through such an ordeal.

Just as the doctor said would happen, they began the five-day steroid treatment for the limbic encephalitis. The test results to confirm this diagnosis would not be in until a couple of weeks, and time was crucial for this disease. Time would be key in his recovery. Hopefully, this could help Jose. I stood with him until all the tests had been completed and the IV containing the steroid therapy had begun. He was ready to rest, as it had been a rough day. He did not understand what was going on, but that's what I was there for – to help

The Quiet Storm

him out.

I knew he was truly sick because, when I left the hospital that day at midnight, he never called me to see if I got home okay. This hurt me so much, but I knew that this was not his normal self.

Good night, my love, I shall see you tomorrow. I know how much you love me. You have made that apparent in all the 30 years we have been together. "Duerme con los Angelitos," I would say to Jose in Spanish when I would leave his hospital room at the end of my visit. This means, "Sleep with the Angels." Then I would add, "But don't forget to come back."

I love the winter, and this winter snowed like no other. Leaving Jose at the end of the visit was so painful, like nothing I had ever experienced before. The lonely feeling as I walked the long stretch of corridor that leads to the elevator, to

The Quiet Storm

standing at the bus stop and arriving to an empty home was more than I could bare. My sister Maria always called me to see how Jose was doing and to ensure that I'd made it home safe.

It had been one week since Jose had admitted, and the steroid treatment for limbic encephalitis began; we now were looking forward to him being discharged. That morning, I received a telephone call from Dr. Yoo informing me that the steroid treatment had not worked as anticipated. She wanted to start him on IVIG infusion. This treatment would last another five days. He would be weaned off the steroids and, at the same time, start the IVIG infusion.

This was not a pleasant experience by any means, but it was necessary, and it was not time to start acting like babies. We took the news as well as anyone could and started the next round of therapy with hope. I noticed during this admission, that Jose was always talking about his mother. He would tell me that she had been there with him and he was laying on her lap. I would often remind him that his mom had died, and it was as if I were delivering this news to him for the first time every time.

Finally, Jose was released after two weeks of being in the hospital and undergoing an enormous amount of testing and therapy. It was nearing his 55th birthday, and we were so happy he was going home at last. He'd often felt that he would never go home again. I imagine that was a scary thought. Hopefully, we thought, this would be the end of the hospitalizations.

The Quiet Storm

CHAPTER 9

As is customary with such a severe disease, Jose would always have to follow up with the neurologist shortly after his discharge from the hospital. This time, he met with his neurologist two weeks after being released. The doctor would perform another MOCA evaluation on him and then send him to the lab to check the Voltage Gated Potassium Antibody Channels. Screening for the antibody protein responsible for the inflammation in his brain would be an ongoing process.

Two weeks after this visit, one of the doctors that worked with the main neurologist called me to get an insight as to how Jose was doing. There were not many positive things to share with her, as I felt there were no significant improvements. The

66

The Quiet Storm

doctor would arrange for him to be admitted once again in about one week. Admission was set for April 17, 2014.

It seemed like he was being hospitalized at least once a month. Upon admission, they would set him up on the brain monitor and perform neurological tests to see if he was improving. He would be scheduled once more for the IVIG infusion. After this discharge, I felt like he had improved this time.

I noticed that he was remembering more details and seemed alert. He was also looking very handsome as well, but according to the doctor, the inflammation had decreased, "not much."

I had decided that I needed to let him be as normal as possible. I could not start caring for him as you would an 80-year-old. He seemed to be getting better, but how much better was anybody's

The Quiet Storm

guess. At the start of this disease, I was scared to death. Would this end his life at a faster rate? Would he turn violent? I didn't know anyone with this particular situation, so I had nothing to compare it to.

The only person I knew with a similar case was my cousin's daughter who had become infected with encephalitis when they'd visited Walt Disney World over ten years before. She was very young at the time, about six years old, when she became bedridden due to her encephalitis. She had contracted the viral type and ended up developing a real severe case of it. It took her about a year to recover as her health got so bad she was not able to get up from bed. She had to learn to walk, talk, eat, and dress again. I remember how my cousin held nightly prayer vigils. I imagine that he could not believe what had happened to him either.

Sometimes, now, I try to peek at Jose through the side of my eye to see how he is acting, to see if he seems okay. My first instinct is to accompany him wherever he goes, but that is not realistic and very exhausting. If I did that, I would not allow him to exercise his judgment, so I must stay put and allow him to continue life as normal as possible. I guess as time goes by and I see improvement, I will feel better about letting him going out on his own.

Allowing him to assert his independence is frightening. I call him continuously to ensure that he is where he is supposed to be. Sometimes, when he steps away, I try to read a little more about what he is suffering. I try to learn about limbic encephalitis while maintaining my composure so I do not break down in front of him. I have my sisters for that.

The Quiet Storm

Once again, it was time to see the Neurologist to check on how Jose had improved since his treatment was administered in the hospital on April 2014. I thought he was doing okay, but as we were sitting at the doctor's office, all of a sudden, he showed a different side of himself that I had not seen.

During his conversation with her, he seemed vulnerable and began to tell her that he was not feeling well at all. He told her that he was so confused, that sometimes he didn't not know if he were coming or going. He told her that he was also experiencing a lot of headaches. The doctor seemed to think that it was due to the Topamax and, therefore, gave him a new prescription with details on how to wean off the medication. During our visit, the doctor asked him to draw a clock, and his brain was so out of it that he didn't want to do it. He was not having a good evaluation day.

The Quiet Storm

Dr. Yoo recommended that Jose have rituximab therapy. She explained that this therapy is used to treat certain types of cancer. Apparently, the bad evaluation from today, combined with the blood test done previously, indicated that the encephalitis was getting worse. He needed a more aggressive approach to be taken.

This threw me for I loop – I had noticed an improvement; however, doctors have their way to assess where a patient is with regards to their memory and cognitive skills by performing a MOCA Evaluation. When we got home, I tried to test him to see if he would be able to draw the clock for me. He drew a clock, but it was backwards. The only thing that was correct was the 12 and the 6. The 1-5 numbers were placed where the 11-7 numbers should be. Apparently something was still wrong.

The Quiet Storm

May 19 and June 2, 2014

The Rituxan therapy had not been approved to be done on an outside basis. Jose's insurance company wanted the treatment to be done as inpatient care, so he had to go to the hospital to get his Rituxan treatment on two separate occasions.

At last, both Rituxan treatments were administered without any immediate side effects, other than standard issues such as an allergic reaction. As part of the treatment, steroids were also given before the Rituxan was to be administered. Two treatments of Rituxan was considered to be complete.

Jose was feeling great after the Rituxan treatment; however, about one week after the last Rituxan treatment, Jose began to experience extreme chills and nausea around the clock; one attack about every 15 minutes. Jose was also getting pains in the right side of his ribs. I was worried because I wanted to ensure that his organs were not being compromised. Rituxan is a relatively new treatment, and all the long term side effects are not fully understood. He had been doing so well, that I was sure that this would be it. Usually, these little bumps in the limbic encephalitis road indicated that a hospitalization would be necessary. The doctor felt that these chills might be a warning that he was having seizures, so once again, she arranged for him to be hospitalized.

The Quiet Storm

June 23, 2014

Hospitalizations are usually so hard on us – the emotion, the sadness, and the idea of how this will eventually end is mentally gripping. My mom is going through Alzheimer's/Dementia and is not doing well herself. Apparently, she is going through a totally different set of neurological issues herself. As if I am not saddened enough already, my mom's situation is so hurtful to me, as I do not see her situation getting any better.

I deal with her issues and oversee all her medical care. I also ensure that my mom's medications are placed in her dispenser so she can take them as directed. I try to be there for her as much as I can to help her as she too needs my help.

Hospitalization day came, and as was

customary, I took Jose to the department of admission so that he could be hospitalized. This hospital stay was to last 2–3 days. The doctor wanted Jose on the brain monitor to check if he was still having seizures.

When Jose went in for his hospital stay, he was in such a good mood, but as the days went by, he became agitated, as they had not yet put the Brain Monitor on him. It took about two days before they would finally place him on the monitor. The next day, the doctor called to let me know that Jose had had seizures from 2:00 AM until about 9:00 AM – he'd had one seizure every hour. He would be given a Dilantin load and then placed back on his regular medications. In addition, they would also start him on a five-day course of IVIG infusion and, upon discharge, set him up to get weekly IVIG infusions for the next three months.

The Quiet Storm

After being released from the hospital, I noticed that he was not feeling well at all. Apparently, the Dilantin load given to him to control the seizures was more than his body could handle. He was not doing well at all; he was more ill upon discharge than when he was admitted. This new medication was not sitting well with him, it seemed. Upon discharge, I let him go to the neurologist on his own, despite the fact that the Dilantin had had an adverse reaction on him. At the neurologist's visit, she wrote down the instructions on how to taper off the Dilantin and re-introduce the Topamax. I was very proud of him for going to his doctor's visit on his own.

Weaning him off and starting a new medication would be done gradually and carefully. He was so eager to be off the Dilantin, but we had to do it by the book. A week after the weaning started, I noticed that he was not feeling well. One night right before bedtime, I noticed that Jose was covered up to his neck and looked very scared – I think paranoia is his "aura." I asked him, "Are you okay?" and he responded, " I am tired of being sick." It looked as if he was trying to hold back the inevitable. Just as he was saying this, he began to have a seizure. I remained calm and held him on his side while calling his name. The seizure was very brief.

I was so devastated about this seizure that I stayed up all night while he rested. I told him that when morning came we were going to the emergency room, which made him very upset. I told him that I would call the neurologist first to see what she recommended. Morning came, and I called Dr. Yoo's office, immediately leaving a message for her to call me back as soon as possible.

The Quiet Storm

When Dr. Yoo called me back, she had told me that there was no need for him to come into the emergency room. She also said that seizures were anticipated when tapering off the Dilantin. I was euphoric because she expressed that she thought Jose was headed in the right direction. Apparently, when he'd gone for his follow-up, he'd had a good evaluation, and his cognitive responses had been much better. She also had reviewed his labs and noticed that his glucose levels had also improved.

During our conversation, I also mentioned to her that, when he'd seen his new primary doctor a couple of days before, the doctor had deemed that one of the high blood pressure medications could be eliminated. She seemed to be pleased with his recent prognosis, as was I.

I fell asleep peacefully that morning. Finally.

The Quiet Storm

Chapter 10

Jose he had been going for IVIG infusions on a weekly basis, just as the doctor had prescribed. I have noticed that he seems a lot better; now when he gets sick or confused, he says, "I can shake it off faster." I guess that means it's not as intense as it used to be. The paranoia episodes that he had experienced during the earlier months, have now gone away as well. Compared to the way this started, I would dare to say it is so much better.

In addition to all the therapy given to Jose such as, Steroids, IVIG Infusion and Rituxan Treatment, Dr. Yoo started Jose on a new regimen of medications called CellCept and Sulfamethazole. This change in medication was definitely needed due to an increase in the antibody titer after Jose's treatment had come to an end.

However, immediately after starting these new

medications, the antibody levels began to decrease. The antibody levels had gone down to zero; its highest point being 731 when all this began. I still worry, though. It's going to be some time before we can say that he is cured, and of course, there is always a chance of a relapse.

I think that this whole nightmare of Jose getting this rare disease has done something to my psyche. From time to time, when I am alone, no matter where I am at, I begin to think about everything I have been through; Jose's suffering makes me tear up, and I become very emotional. I think I have been traumatized.

I kiss and hug Jose every day, so many times, one cannot count. I ensure that I treat him like a king. If he were to die tomorrow from this rare disease, he could honestly say, "My wife truly did love me," and I would respond, "Que duermas con los Angelitos."

The Quiet Storm

It is said that people with this type of disease often mention seeing their dead loved ones. Does the mind take you to a place of piece and comfort when you are at your worst or does this mean that your loved ones, who have passed away, actually surround you when you are dying? Is it a hallucination?

When I mentioned to Jose about seeing the young man standing behind him in the mirror , he said, "Oh, you saw him too - I thought I was crazy when I felt his presence the other day as I was sleeping and I felt someone hugging me so tight." I said to him, "Easy, you are squeezing me too hard."

Do people who have this disease experience seeing their loved ones who have passed away, or do we all participate in one big hallucination?

The Quiet Storm

For more information on encephalitis go to

www.encephalitis.info

The Quiet Storm

The Quiet Storm

83

The Quiet Storm

www.ingramcontent.com/pod-product-compliance
Lightning Source LLC
Chambersburg PA
CBHW060404190526
45169CB00002B/742